SOMATIC DIET FOR NERVOUS SYSTEM REGULATION

The complete easy way solution to somatic pain, loss up to 20 pounds with 365day delicious recipes plus 14day meal plan to stay fitness.

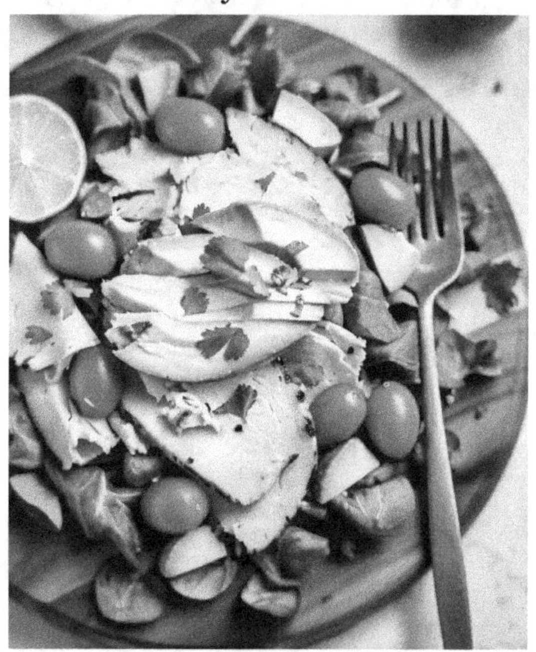

JENNIFER .S COLE

TABLE OF CONTENT

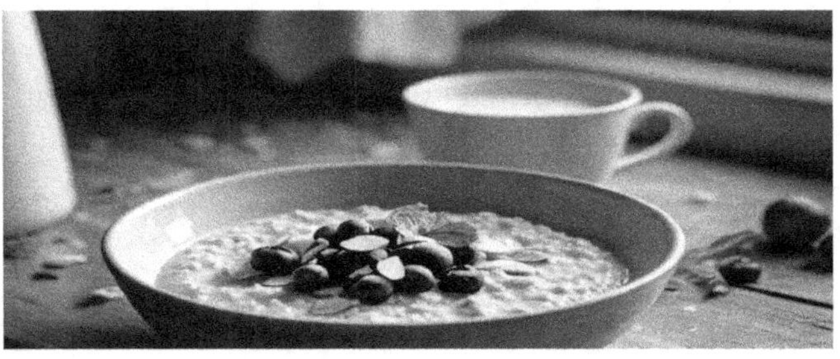

Are you tired of feeling overwhelmed, anxious, or on edge? Do you long for a sense of calm and inner peace, even in the midst of life's daily stressors? If so, the Somatic Diet for Nervous System Regulation offers a powerful solution.

Within the pages of this transformative book, you'll discover a holistic approach to nourishing your body and mind, one that goes beyond simple dietary changes. The somatic diet is a way of life that harmonizes the connection between what you eat and how you feel, promoting balance and regulation in your nervous system.

By embracing whole, nutrient-dense foods and eliminating inflammatory triggers, you'll be taking the first step towards calming dysregulation and restoring your body's natural rhythms. But the somatic diet is about more than just the food on your plate – it's a journey of self-discovery, mindfulness, and gentle movement practices that cultivate a deeper sense of embodiment and self-awareness.

Prepare to unlock the secrets of a regulated nervous system, one bite at a time. With easy-to-follow recipes, practical tips, and invaluable insights, this book will guide you towards a life of greater peace, resilience, and overall well-being.

Say goodbye to the constant state of frazzle and hello to a new era of balance and vitality. The Somatic Diet for Nervous System Regulation is your gateway to a calmer, more centered you.

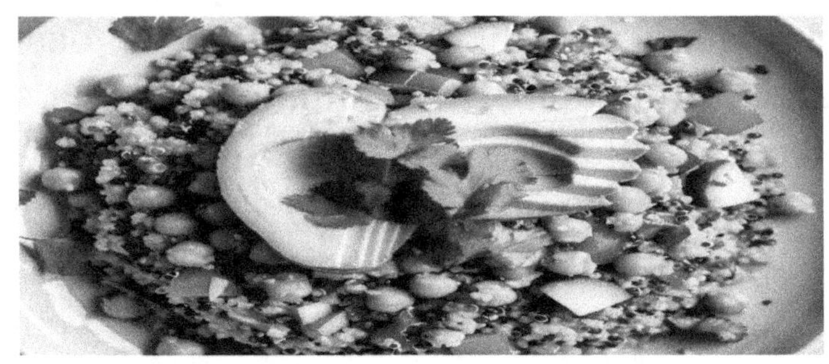

Chapter 1:WHAT IS SOMATIC SYMPTOMS DISORDER?

When a person experiences severe distress and/or functional difficulties as a result of intense concentration on bodily symptoms, such as pain, weakness, or shortness of breath, it is determined that they have somatic symptom disorder. Regarding the physical symptoms, the person exhibits excessive sensations, thoughts, and behaviors. The individual is exhibiting symptoms and thinks they are ill, even if the physical symptoms are not connected to a recognized medical condition (that is, not faking the sickness).

When a medical explanation for a physical symptom cannot be found, a person is not diagnosed with somatic symptom disorder. The focus is on how excessive or out of proportion the illness-related thoughts, feelings, and behaviors are.

Chapter 2:DIAGNOSED?

One or more physically bothersome symptoms that interfere with day-to-day activities

Excessive sentiments, thoughts, or actions associated with at least one of the following in relation to the physical symptoms or health concerns:

persistent thoughts that are excessive for the severity of the symptoms

persistently high concern for one's health or symptoms

Spending too much attention and effort on the symptoms or health issues

At least one symptom is present all the time, though there could be other symptoms as well as intermittent symptoms.

Usually, patients with somatic symptom disorder see a primary care physician instead of a psychiatrist or another mental health specialist. People who suffer from somatic symptom disorder could find it hard to realize that their worries about their symptoms are unwarranted. Even after being presented proof that they do not have a dangerous ailment, they may still feel anxious and afraid. For some people, the primary symptom is pain. By the age of 30, somatic symptom disorders typically start.

Chapter 3:TREATMENT?

The goal of treatment for somatic symptom disorder is to assist manage symptoms and restore as much normalcy to the patient's life as possible.

Typically, treatment for somatic symptom disorder entails routine appointments with a dependable medical provider. In addition to monitoring patient health and symptoms and avoiding pointless tests and treatments, the doctor can provide comfort and support. Through psychotherapy, or talk therapy, a person might acquire new coping mechanisms for pain or other symptoms, manage stress, and enhance functioning.

In the event that the patient additionally suffers from severe anxiety or depression, antidepressant drugs may be helpful.

Chapter 4:RELATED DISORDER?

Anxiety disorder related to illness?

The former term for illness anxiety condition was "hypochondriasis." The individual is consumed with being sick or being sick, and they worry about their health nonstop. They might regularly examine themselves for symptoms of disease and take great care to prevent hazards to their health. An individual with disease anxiety condition typically does not have symptoms, in contrast to somatic symptom disorder.

Disorder of conversion?

When there is no indication of a physical reason, a person with conversion disorder (also known as functional neurological symptom disorder) experiences symptoms that impair their perception, feeling, or mobility. A person might experience difficulties walking, eyesight, or numbness. Usually, the symptoms strike suddenly. The symptoms might not go away right away or they might persist for a while. Anxiety or depression are also common in people with conversion disorder.

Factitious disorder is the deliberate exacerbation of a minor sickness or the production of physical or mental illness in those who are not truly ill. A factitious disorder sufferer may also inflict harm or disease on another person (factitious disorder imposed on another), for example, by pretending to be a youngster in their care. The individual creating the circumstance may or may not appear to gain anything from it (such getting out of work or school).

Chapter 5: BREAKFAST RECIPES

1. Greek Yogurt Parfait

Ingredients:

- 1 cup plain Greek yogurt
- 1/2 cup mixed berries (strawberries, blueberries, raspberries)
- 1/4 cup granola
- 1 tablespoon honey

- 1 tablespoon chia seeds

Instructions:

1. In a glass or bowl, layer half of the Greek yogurt.
2. Add half of the mixed berries.
3. Sprinkle half of the granola on top.
4. Repeat the layers with the remaining yogurt, berries, and granola.
5. Drizzle honey over the top and sprinkle with chia seeds.
6. Serve immediately.

Nutritional Information (per serving):

- Calories: 350
- Protein: 20g
- Carbohydrates: 45g
- Fat: 10g
- Fiber: 6g
- Sugar: 25g

2. **Avocado Toast with Poached Egg**

Ingredients:

- 1 slice whole-grain bread
- 1/2 ripe avocado
- 1 large egg
- 1 teaspoon lemon juice
- Salt and pepper to taste
- Red pepper flakes (optional)

Instructions:

1. Toast the whole-grain bread until golden brown.
2. In a small bowl, mash the avocado with lemon juice, salt, and pepper.
3. Spread the mashed avocado on the toasted bread.
4. Poach the egg: Bring a pot of water to a simmer, create a whirlpool, and gently slide the egg into the center. Cook for 3-4 minutes until the white is set but the yolk is runny.

5. Place the poached egg on top of the avocado toast.
6. Sprinkle with red pepper flakes if desired.
7. Serve immediately.

Nutritional Information (per serving):

- Calories: 280
- Protein: 11g
- Carbohydrates: 24g
- Fat: 18g
- Fiber: 7g
- Sugar: 2g

3. Oatmeal with Fresh Fruit and Nuts

Ingredients:

- 1/2 cup rolled oats
- 1 cup water or milk (dairy or non-dairy)
- 1/2 apple, diced

- 1 tablespoon almond butter
- 1 tablespoon chopped walnuts
- 1 teaspoon cinnamon
- 1 teaspoon honey (optional)

Instructions:

1. In a small pot, bring the water or milk to a boil.
2. Add the rolled oats and reduce the heat to a simmer. Cook for about 5 minutes, stirring occasionally.
3. Once the oats are cooked, transfer to a bowl.
4. Top with diced apple, almond butter, chopped walnuts, and cinnamon.
5. Drizzle with honey if desired.
6. Serve warm.

Nutritional Information (per serving):

- Calories: 350
- Protein: 9g

- Carbohydrates: 52g
- Fat: 14g
- Fiber: 8g
- Sugar: 15g

4. **Spinach and Feta Omelette**

Ingredients:

- 2 large eggs
- 1/2 cup fresh spinach, chopped
- 1/4 cup crumbled feta cheese
- 1 tablespoon olive oil
- Salt and pepper to taste

Instructions:

1. In a bowl, whisk the eggs with a pinch of salt and pepper.
2. Heat the olive oil in a non-stick skillet over medium heat.
3. Add the spinach and sauté until wilted, about 1-2 minutes.

4. Pour the eggs into the skillet, swirling to cover the pan evenly.
5. Cook until the edges start to set, then sprinkle the feta cheese over one half of the omelette.
6. Fold the other half of the omelette over the cheese and cook for another minute until the eggs are fully set.
7. Serve immediately.

Nutritional Information (per serving):

- Calories: 250
- Protein: 15g
- Carbohydrates: 3g
- Fat: 20g
- Fiber: 1g
- Sugar: 1g

5. Smoothie Bowl

Ingredients:

- 1 frozen banana
- 1/2 cup frozen mixed berries
- 1/2 cup spinach
- 1/2 cup unsweetened almond milk
- 1 tablespoon chia seeds
- 1 tablespoon almond butter
- 1/4 cup granola (for topping)

Instructions:

1. In a blender, combine the frozen banana, frozen berries, spinach, almond milk, chia seeds, and almond butter. Blend until smooth and thick.
2. Pour the smoothie into a bowl.
3. Top with granola and additional fresh fruit if desired.
4. Serve immediately with a spoon.

Nutritional Information (per serving):

- Calories: 350
- Protein: 8g

- Carbohydrates: 52g
- Fat: 14g
- Fiber: 10g
- Sugar: 25g

1. **Quinoa Salad with Chickpeas and Avocado**

Ingredients:

- 1 cup cooked quinoa
- 1/2 cup canned chickpeas, drained and rinsed
- 1 avocado, diced
- 1/2 cup cherry tomatoes, halved
- 1/4 cup red onion, finely chopped
- 1/4 cup fresh cilantro, chopped
- 2 tablespoons olive oil
- 1 tablespoon lemon juice
- Salt and pepper to taste

Instructions:

1. In a large bowl, combine cooked quinoa, chickpeas, avocado, cherry tomatoes, red onion, and cilantro.
2. In a small bowl, whisk together olive oil, lemon juice, salt, and pepper.
3. Pour the dressing over the quinoa mixture and toss to combine.
4. Serve chilled or at room temperature.

Nutritional Information (per serving):

- Calories: 400
- Protein: 10g
- Carbohydrates: 45g
- Fat: 22g
- Fiber: 12g
- Sugar: 4g

2. Grilled Chicken and Vegetable Wrap

Ingredients:

- 1 whole-grain tortilla
- 4 oz grilled chicken breast, sliced
- 1/2 cup mixed grilled vegetables (bell peppers, zucchini, onions)
- 1/4 cup hummus
- 1/4 cup fresh spinach leaves

Instructions:

1. Spread hummus evenly over the tortilla.
2. Layer with grilled chicken, mixed grilled vegetables, and spinach leaves.
3. Roll up the tortilla tightly and slice in half.
4. Serve immediately or wrap in foil for later.

Nutritional Information (per serving):

- Calories: 350
- Protein: 28g

- Carbohydrates: 35g
- Fat: 12g
- Fiber: 8g
- Sugar: 4g

3. Lentil Soup

Ingredients:

- 1 cup dried lentils, rinsed
- 1 carrot, diced
- 1 celery stalk, diced
- 1 small onion, diced
- 2 garlic cloves, minced
- 4 cups vegetable broth
- 1 can (14.5 oz) diced tomatoes
- 1 teaspoon cumin
- 1 teaspoon paprika
- 1 tablespoon olive oil
- Salt and pepper to taste

Instructions:

1. Heat olive oil in a large pot over medium heat. Add onion, carrot, and celery, and cook until softened, about 5 minutes.
2. Add garlic, cumin, and paprika, and cook for another minute.
3. Add lentils, vegetable broth, and diced tomatoes. Bring to a boil.
4. Reduce heat and simmer for 30-40 minutes, or until lentils are tender.
5. Season with salt and pepper to taste.
6. Serve hot.

Nutritional Information (per serving):

- Calories: 250
- Protein: 15g
- Carbohydrates: 40g
- Fat: 5g
- Fiber: 15g
- Sugar: 8g

4. Turkey and Avocado Salad

Ingredients:

- 2 cups mixed greens (spinach, arugula, romaine)
- 4 oz sliced turkey breast
- 1 avocado, diced
- 1/2 cup cherry tomatoes, halved
- 1/4 cup red onion, thinly sliced
- 1 tablespoon olive oil
- 1 tablespoon balsamic vinegar
- Salt and pepper to taste

Instructions:

1. In a large bowl, combine mixed greens, turkey breast, avocado, cherry tomatoes, and red onion.
2. In a small bowl, whisk together olive oil, balsamic vinegar, salt, and pepper.
3. Drizzle the dressing over the salad and toss to combine.
4. Serve immediately.

Nutritional Information (per serving):

- Calories: 350
- Protein: 24g
- Carbohydrates: 15g
- Fat: 24g
- Fiber: 10g
- Sugar: 5g

5. **Stuffed Bell Peppers**

Ingredients:

- 2 large bell peppers, halved and seeds removed
- 1 cup cooked brown rice
- 1/2 cup black beans, drained and rinsed
- 1/2 cup corn kernels
- 1/4 cup diced tomatoes
- 1/4 cup shredded cheddar cheese
- 1 tablespoon olive oil
- 1 teaspoon chili powder
- 1 teaspoon cumin

- Salt and pepper to taste

Instructions:

1. Preheat oven to 375°F (190°C).
2. In a large bowl, combine cooked brown rice, black beans, corn, diced tomatoes, olive oil, chili powder, cumin, salt, and pepper.
3. Stuff the bell pepper halves with the rice mixture and place them in a baking dish.
4. Top each stuffed pepper with shredded cheddar cheese.
5. Cover with foil and bake for 30 minutes. Remove the foil and bake for an additional 10 minutes, until the cheese is melted and bubbly.
6. Serve hot.

Nutritional Information (per serving):

- Calories: 300

- Protein: 10g
- Carbohydrates: 45g
- Fat: 10g
- Fiber: 10g
- Sugar: 8g

Chapter 7: DINNER RECIPES

1. **Baked Salmon with Quinoa and Asparagus**

Ingredients:

- 4 salmon fillets (4 oz each)
- 1 cup quinoa, rinsed
- 2 cups water or vegetable broth
- 1 bunch asparagus, trimmed
- 2 tablespoons olive oil
- 2 tablespoons lemon juice
- 1 teaspoon garlic powder
- Salt and pepper to taste

Instructions:

1. Preheat the oven to 400°F (200°C).
2. Place the salmon fillets on a baking sheet lined with parchment paper. Drizzle with 1 tablespoon olive oil, 1 tablespoon lemon juice, garlic powder, salt, and pepper.
3. Arrange the asparagus around the salmon. Drizzle with remaining olive oil, lemon juice, salt, and pepper.
4. Bake for 15-20 minutes, or until the salmon is cooked through and flakes easily with a fork.
5. Meanwhile, bring 2 cups of water or vegetable broth to a boil in a medium pot. Add quinoa, reduce heat to low, cover, and simmer for 15 minutes, or until the quinoa is cooked and the liquid is absorbed.
6. Serve the baked salmon with quinoa and asparagus.

Nutritional Information (per serving):

- Calories: 450
- Protein: 35g
- Carbohydrates: 30g
- Fat: 20g
- Fiber: 5g
- Sugar: 2g

2. Chicken Stir-Fry with Brown Rice

Ingredients:

- 2 boneless, skinless chicken breasts, sliced into thin strips
- 1 cup brown rice, cooked
- 2 cups mixed vegetables (bell peppers, broccoli, snap peas, carrots)
- 2 tablespoons soy sauce (or tamari for gluten-free)
- 1 tablespoon olive oil
- 1 teaspoon sesame oil
- 2 garlic cloves, minced
- 1 teaspoon fresh ginger, grated
- 1 tablespoon sesame seeds (optional)

- Salt and pepper to taste

Instructions:

1. Heat olive oil in a large skillet or wok over medium-high heat.
2. Add garlic and ginger, and cook for 1 minute until fragrant.
3. Add chicken strips and cook until no longer pink, about 5-7 minutes.
4. Add mixed vegetables and cook for another 5-7 minutes until tender-crisp.
5. Stir in soy sauce, sesame oil, salt, and pepper.
6. Serve the stir-fry over cooked brown rice, garnished with sesame seeds if desired.

Nutritional Information (per serving):

- Calories: 400
- Protein: 30g

- Carbohydrates: 45g
- Fat: 12g
- Fiber: 6g
- Sugar: 4g

3. Vegetable Curry with Chickpeas

Ingredients:

- 1 can (15 oz) chickpeas, drained and rinsed
- 1 cup coconut milk
- 1 cup vegetable broth
- 2 cups mixed vegetables (cauliflower, bell peppers, carrots, spinach)
- 1 onion, diced
- 2 garlic cloves, minced
- 1 tablespoon curry powder
- 1 teaspoon cumin
- 1 tablespoon olive oil
- Salt and pepper to taste
- Fresh cilantro for garnish

Instructions:

1. Heat olive oil in a large pot over medium heat.
2. Add onion and garlic, and cook until soft, about 5 minutes.
3. Stir in curry powder and cumin, and cook for another minute.
4. Add chickpeas, mixed vegetables, coconut milk, and vegetable broth. Bring to a boil.
5. Reduce heat and simmer for 20-25 minutes, until vegetables are tender.
6. Season with salt and pepper to taste.
7. Garnish with fresh cilantro and serve with rice or naan.

Nutritional Information (per serving):

- Calories: 350
- Protein: 10g
- Carbohydrates: 45g
- Fat: 16g
- Fiber: 10g

- Sugar: 8g

4. Turkey Meatballs with Zucchini Noodles

Ingredients:

- 1 lb ground turkey
- 1/4 cup breadcrumbs (or almond flour for gluten-free)
- 1/4 cup grated Parmesan cheese
- 1 egg, beaten
- 2 garlic cloves, minced
- 1 teaspoon dried oregano
- Salt and pepper to taste
- 2 tablespoons olive oil
- 4 zucchinis, spiralized
- 1 cup marinara sauce

Instructions:

1. In a large bowl, combine ground turkey, breadcrumbs, Parmesan

cheese, egg, garlic, oregano, salt, and pepper. Mix until well combined.

2. Form the mixture into 12-16 meatballs.
3. Heat 1 tablespoon olive oil in a large skillet over medium heat. Add meatballs and cook until browned on all sides and cooked through, about 10-12 minutes.
4. Remove meatballs from skillet and set aside.
5. In the same skillet, heat the remaining olive oil and add zucchini noodles. Cook for 2-3 minutes until slightly softened.
6. Add marinara sauce and meatballs to the skillet, and stir to combine. Cook for another 2-3 minutes until heated through.
7. Serve immediately.

Nutritional Information (per serving):

- Calories: 400

- Protein: 30g
- Carbohydrates: 20g
- Fat: 20g
- Fiber: 5g
- Sugar: 8g

5. Beef and Broccoli Stir-Fry

Ingredients:

- 1 lb flank steak, thinly sliced
- 2 cups broccoli florets
- 1 bell pepper, sliced
- 1/4 cup soy sauce (or tamari for gluten-free)
- 2 tablespoons oyster sauce
- 1 tablespoon cornstarch
- 1 tablespoon olive oil
- 1 teaspoon sesame oil
- 2 garlic cloves, minced
- 1 teaspoon fresh ginger, grated
- Cooked brown rice for serving

Instructions:

1. In a small bowl, mix soy sauce, oyster sauce, and cornstarch. Add beef slices and marinate for 15 minutes.
2. Heat olive oil in a large skillet or wok over medium-high heat.
3. Add garlic and ginger, and cook for 1 minute until fragrant.
4. Add marinated beef and cook until browned, about 5-7 minutes.
5. Add broccoli and bell pepper, and cook for another 5-7 minutes until tender-crisp.
6. Drizzle with sesame oil and stir to combine.
7. Serve over cooked brown rice.

Nutritional Information (per serving):

- Calories: 450
- Protein: 35g
- Carbohydrates: 40g
- Fat: 15g

- Fiber: 6g
- Sugar: 6g

Chapter 8:DESSERT RECIPES

1. Dark Chocolate Avocado Mousse

Ingredients:

- 2 ripe avocados
- 1/2 cup unsweetened cocoa powder
- 1/2 cup maple syrup or honey
- 1/4 cup almond milk
- 1 teaspoon vanilla extract
- Pinch of salt

Instructions:

1. Cut the avocados in half, remove the pits, and scoop the flesh into a food processor.
2. Add cocoa powder, maple syrup, almond milk, vanilla extract, and salt.

3. Blend until smooth and creamy.

4. Spoon the mousse into serving dishes and chill for at least 30 minutes before serving.

Nutritional Information (per serving):

- Calories: 250
- Protein: 3g
- Carbohydrates: 36g
- Fat: 14g
- Fiber: 7g
- Sugar: 22g

2. Berry Chia Pudding

Ingredients:

- 1 cup unsweetened almond milk
- 1/4 cup chia seeds
- 1 tablespoon maple syrup or honey
- 1/2 teaspoon vanilla extract

- 1 cup mixed berries (strawberries, blueberries, raspberries)

Instructions:

1. In a bowl, whisk together almond milk, chia seeds, maple syrup, and vanilla extract.
2. Let the mixture sit for 5 minutes, then whisk again to prevent clumping.
3. Cover and refrigerate for at least 4 hours or overnight until the pudding thickens.
4. Before serving, top with mixed berries.

Nutritional Information (per serving):

- Calories: 200
- Protein: 4g
- Carbohydrates: 27g
- Fat: 10g
- Fiber: 10g
- Sugar: 13g

3. **Baked Apples with Cinnamon and Walnuts**

Ingredients:

- 4 large apples
- 1/4 cup chopped walnuts
- 2 tablespoons maple syrup or honey
- 1 teaspoon ground cinnamon
- 1/2 teaspoon ground nutmeg
- 1 tablespoon coconut oil

Instructions:

1. Preheat the oven to 375°F (190°C).
2. Core the apples, leaving the bottoms intact.
3. In a small bowl, mix together walnuts, maple syrup, cinnamon, nutmeg, and coconut oil.
4. Stuff the mixture into the cored apples.
5. Place the apples in a baking dish and cover with foil.

6. Bake for 20 minutes, then remove the foil and bake for an additional 10-15 minutes until the apples are tender.
7. Serve warm.

Nutritional Information (per serving):

- Calories: 200
- Protein: 2g
- Carbohydrates: 34g
- Fat: 8g
- Fiber: 6g
- Sugar: 24g

4. Greek Yogurt and Honey Tart

Ingredients:

- 1 cup Greek yogurt
- 2 tablespoons honey
- 1 teaspoon vanilla extract
- 1 premade graham cracker crust (9 inches)

- Fresh fruit for topping (strawberries, blueberries, kiwi)

Instructions:

1. In a bowl, mix Greek yogurt, honey, and vanilla extract until well combined.
2. Pour the mixture into the graham cracker crust and spread evenly.
3. Top with fresh fruit of your choice.
4. Chill in the refrigerator for at least 1 hour before serving.

Nutritional Information (per serving):

- Calories: 220
- Protein: 6g
- Carbohydrates: 36g
- Fat: 7g
- Fiber: 2g
- Sugar: 20g

5. Coconut Macaroons

Ingredients:

- 2 cups unsweetened shredded coconut
- 1/2 cup sweetened condensed milk
- 1 teaspoon vanilla extract
- 2 large egg whites
- 1/4 teaspoon salt

Instructions:

1. Preheat the oven to 325°F (165°C) and line a baking sheet with parchment paper.
2. In a large bowl, mix together shredded coconut, sweetened condensed milk, and vanilla extract.
3. In a separate bowl, beat the egg whites and salt until stiff peaks form.
4. Gently fold the egg whites into the coconut mixture.

5. Using a tablespoon, drop small mounds of the mixture onto the prepared baking sheet.
6. Bake for 20-25 minutes, or until the macaroons are golden brown.
7. Let cool before serving.

Nutritional Information (per serving):

- Calories: 150
- Protein: 2g
- Carbohydrates: 18g
- Fat: 8g
- Fiber: 2g
- Sugar: 15g

Chapter 9: SNACKS RECIPES

1. Homemade Trail Mix

Ingredients:

- 1 cup mixed nuts (almonds, cashews, peanuts)
- 1/2 cup dried fruits (raisins, cranberries, apricots)
- 1/4 cup dark chocolate chips
- 1/4 cup pumpkin seeds (optional)

Instructions:

1. In a bowl, combine mixed nuts, dried fruits, dark chocolate chips, and pumpkin seeds.
2. Mix well.
3. Store in an airtight container for up to one week.

Nutritional Information (per serving):

- Calories: 200
- Protein: 5g
- Carbohydrates: 20g
- Fat: 12g
- Fiber: 3g

- Sugar: 12g

2. Greek Yogurt with Berries

Ingredients:

- 1 cup Greek yogurt
- 1/2 cup mixed berries (strawberries, blueberries, raspberries)
- 1 tablespoon honey (optional)

Instructions:

1. In a bowl, spoon Greek yogurt.
2. Top with mixed berries.
3. Drizzle with honey if desired.

Nutritional Information (per serving):

- Calories: 150
- Protein: 15g
- Carbohydrates: 20g

- Fat: 0g
- Fiber: 3g
- Sugar: 15g

3. Cucumber Hummus Bites

Ingredients:

- 1 large cucumber
- 1/2 cup hummus
- Cherry tomatoes, sliced (optional)
- Fresh parsley, chopped (optional)

Instructions:

1. Slice the cucumber into rounds.
2. Spoon a small amount of hummus onto each cucumber round.
3. Top with sliced cherry tomatoes and chopped parsley if desired.

Nutritional Information (per serving):

- Calories: 50
- Protein: 2g
- Carbohydrates: 6g
- Fat: 2g
- Fiber: 2g
- Sugar: 1g

4. Apple Slices with Almond Butter

Ingredients:

- 1 apple, sliced
- 2 tablespoons almond butter

Instructions:

1. Slice the apple into wedges.
2. Spread almond butter on each apple slice.
3. Serve immediately.

Nutritional Information (per serving):

- Calories: 200
- Protein: 4g
- Carbohydrates: 25g
- Fat: 12g
- Fiber: 6g
- Sugar: 18g

5. **Roasted Chickpeas**

Ingredients:

- 1 can (15 oz) chickpeas, drained and rinsed
- 1 tablespoon olive oil
- 1 teaspoon ground cumin
- 1/2 teaspoon smoked paprika
- 1/2 teaspoon garlic powder
- Salt to taste

Instructions:

1. Preheat the oven to 400°F (200°C).

2. Pat the chickpeas dry with a paper towel and remove any loose skins.
3. In a bowl, toss chickpeas with olive oil, cumin, paprika, garlic powder, and salt.
4. Spread chickpeas in a single layer on a baking sheet lined with parchment paper.
5. Bake for 20-30 minutes, stirring halfway through, until crispy.
6. Let cool before serving.

Nutritional Information (per serving):

- Calories: 150
- Protein: 6g
- Carbohydrates: 20g
- Fat: 5g
- Fiber: 6g
- Sugar: 4g

1. Stuffed Bell Peppers

Ingredients:

- 2 large bell peppers, halved and seeds removed
- 1 cup cooked quinoa
- 1/2 cup black beans, drained and rinsed
- 1/2 cup diced tomatoes
- 1/4 cup diced red onion
- 1/4 cup shredded cheddar cheese
- 1 tablespoon olive oil
- 1 teaspoon cumin
- 1 teaspoon chili powder
- Salt and pepper to taste

Instructions:

1. Preheat the oven to 375°F (190°C).

2. In a skillet, heat olive oil over medium heat. Add diced onion and cook until translucent.

3. Add cooked quinoa, black beans, diced tomatoes, cumin, chili powder, salt, and pepper to the skillet. Cook for 5 minutes until heated through.

4. Spoon the quinoa mixture into the bell pepper halves.

5. Sprinkle shredded cheddar cheese on top of each pepper.

6. Place the stuffed bell peppers on a baking sheet and bake for 20-25 minutes until the peppers are tender and the cheese is melted.

7. Serve hot.

Nutritional Information (per serving):

- Calories: 180
- Protein: 7g
- Carbohydrates: 22g
- Fat: 7g
- Fiber: 6g

- Sugar: 3g

2. Mango Avocado Salsa with Whole Grain Tortilla Chips

Ingredients:

- 1 ripe mango, diced
- 1 ripe avocado, diced
- 1/4 cup red onion, finely chopped
- 1/4 cup fresh cilantro, chopped
- 1 jalapeño, seeded and minced
- 1 lime, juiced
- Salt and pepper to taste
- Whole grain tortilla chips for serving

Instructions:

1. In a bowl, combine diced mango, diced avocado, chopped red onion, chopped cilantro, minced jalapeño, lime juice, salt, and pepper. Mix well.

2. Taste and adjust seasoning if needed.

3. Serve the mango avocado salsa with whole grain tortilla chips.

Nutritional Information (per serving):

- Calories: 120
- Protein: 2g
- Carbohydrates: 18g
- Fat: 6g
- Fiber: 5g
- Sugar: 8g

3. Greek Yogurt Veggie Dip

Ingredients:

- 1 cup plain Greek yogurt
- 1/2 cup grated cucumber
- 1/4 cup grated carrot
- 2 tablespoons chopped fresh dill
- 1 tablespoon lemon juice
- 1 clove garlic, minced

- Salt and pepper to taste
- Assorted raw vegetables for dipping (carrot sticks, cucumber slices, bell pepper strips)

Instructions:

1. In a bowl, combine Greek yogurt, grated cucumber, grated carrot, chopped fresh dill, lemon juice, minced garlic, salt, and pepper. Mix well.
2. Taste and adjust seasoning if needed.
3. Chill the dip in the refrigerator for at least 30 minutes before serving.
4. Serve the Greek yogurt veggie dip with assorted raw vegetables for dipping.

Nutritional Information (per serving, dip only):

- Calories: 60
- Protein: 6g

- Carbohydrates: 6g
- Fat: 1g
- Fiber: 1g
- Sugar: 4g

4. Baked Zucchini Fries

Ingredients:

- 2 medium zucchinis, cut into fries
- 1/2 cup whole wheat breadcrumbs
- 1/4 cup grated Parmesan cheese
- 1 teaspoon garlic powder
- 1 teaspoon dried oregano
- 1/2 teaspoon paprika
- Salt and pepper to taste
- 1 large egg, beaten
- Cooking spray

Instructions:

1. Preheat the oven to 425°F (220°C). Line a baking sheet with parchment

paper and lightly coat with cooking spray.

2. In a shallow dish, combine whole wheat breadcrumbs, grated Parmesan cheese, garlic powder, dried oregano, paprika, salt, and pepper.
3. Dip each zucchini fry into the beaten egg, then coat it with the breadcrumb mixture.
4. Place the coated zucchini fries on the prepared baking sheet in a single layer.
5. Bake for 20-25 minutes, flipping halfway through, until golden and crispy.
6. Serve hot with a side of marinara sauce for dipping.

Nutritional Information (per serving):

- Calories: 100
- Protein: 6g
- Carbohydrates: 12g
- Fat: 4g

- Fiber: 3g
- Sugar: 3g

5. **Caprese Skewers**

Ingredients:

- Cherry tomatoes
- Fresh mozzarella balls
- Fresh basil leaves
- Balsamic glaze
- Toothpicks or small skewers

Instructions:

1. Thread one cherry tomato, one mozzarella ball, and one fresh basil leaf onto each toothpick or small skewer.
2. Arrange the skewers on a serving platter.
3. Drizzle with balsamic glaze before serving.

Nutritional Information (per serving, 3 skewers):

- Calories: 100
- Protein: 6g
- Carbohydrates: 3g
- Fat: 7g
- Fiber: 1g
- Sugar: 2g

1. Vegetable Lentil Soup

Ingredients:

- 1 tablespoon olive oil
- 1 onion, diced
- 2 carrots, diced
- 2 celery stalks, diced
- 2 cloves garlic, minced
- 1 cup dry green lentils, rinsed
- 4 cups vegetable broth
- 1 can (14.5 oz) diced tomatoes

- 2 cups chopped spinach or kale
- 1 teaspoon dried thyme
- Salt and pepper to taste

Instructions:

1. Heat olive oil in a large pot over medium heat. Add diced onion, carrots, and celery. Cook until softened, about 5 minutes.
2. Add minced garlic and cook for another minute.
3. Add dry lentils, vegetable broth, diced tomatoes (with juices), dried thyme, salt, and pepper. Bring to a boil.
4. Reduce heat to low, cover, and simmer for 20-25 minutes, or until lentils are tender.
5. Stir in chopped spinach or kale and cook for an additional 5 minutes until wilted.
6. Adjust seasoning if needed and serve hot.

Nutritional Information (per serving):

- Calories: 250
- Protein: 14g
- Carbohydrates: 40g
- Fat: 4g
- Fiber: 15g
- Sugar: 6g

2. Chicken and Vegetable Soup

Ingredients:

- 1 tablespoon olive oil
- 1 onion, diced
- 2 carrots, diced
- 2 celery stalks, diced
- 2 cloves garlic, minced
- 6 cups chicken broth
- 2 cups cooked shredded chicken breast
- 1 cup diced tomatoes
- 1 cup chopped green beans
- 1 teaspoon dried thyme

- Salt and pepper to taste

Instructions:

1. Heat olive oil in a large pot over medium heat. Add diced onion, carrots, and celery. Cook until softened, about 5 minutes.
2. Add minced garlic and cook for another minute.
3. Pour in chicken broth and bring to a simmer.
4. Add cooked shredded chicken, diced tomatoes, chopped green beans, dried thyme, salt, and pepper. Simmer for 15-20 minutes, until vegetables are tender.
5. Adjust seasoning if needed and serve hot.

Nutritional Information (per serving):

- Calories: 200

- Protein: 20g
- Carbohydrates: 10g
- Fat: 8g
- Fiber: 3g
- Sugar: 4g

3. Beef and Barley Stew

Ingredients:

- 1 tablespoon olive oil
- 1 lb stewing beef, cut into bite-sized pieces
- 1 onion, diced
- 2 carrots, diced
- 2 celery stalks, diced
- 2 cloves garlic, minced
- 4 cups beef broth
- 1 cup water
- 1/2 cup pearl barley
- 1 teaspoon dried thyme
- Salt and pepper to taste

Instructions:

1. Heat olive oil in a large pot over medium-high heat. Add stewing beef and cook until browned on all sides, about 5 minutes.
2. Add diced onion, carrots, and celery. Cook until softened, about 5 minutes.
3. Add minced garlic and cook for another minute.
4. Pour in beef broth and water. Bring to a boil.
5. Stir in pearl barley and dried thyme. Reduce heat to low, cover, and simmer for 1 hour, or until beef is tender and barley is cooked.
6. Season with salt and pepper to taste before serving.

Nutritional Information (per serving):

- Calories: 300
- Protein: 25g
- Carbohydrates: 20g

- Fat: 12g
- Fiber: 5g
- Sugar: 3g

4. **Tomato Basil Soup**

Ingredients:

- 1 tablespoon olive oil
- 1 onion, diced
- 2 cloves garlic, minced
- 2 cans (14.5 oz each) diced tomatoes
- 2 cups vegetable broth
- 1/2 cup fresh basil leaves, chopped
- 1/4 cup heavy cream (optional)
- Salt and pepper to taste

Instructions:

1. Heat olive oil in a large pot over medium heat. Add diced onion and cook until softened, about 5 minutes.

2. Add minced garlic and cook for another minute.
3. Pour in diced tomatoes (with juices) and vegetable broth. Bring to a boil.
4. Reduce heat to low and simmer for 15-20 minutes.
5. Stir in chopped basil leaves and heavy cream (if using). Simmer for another 5 minutes.
6. Use an immersion blender to blend the soup until smooth. Alternatively, transfer the soup to a blender and blend until smooth.
7. Season with salt and pepper to taste before serving.

Nutritional Information (per serving):

- Calories: 150
- Protein: 4g
- Carbohydrates: 20g
- Fat: 7g
- Fiber: 5g
- Sugar: 10g

5. **Butternut Squash and Apple Soup**

Ingredients:

- 1 tablespoon olive oil
- 1 onion, diced
- 2 cloves garlic, minced
- 1 butternut squash, peeled, seeded, and cubed
- 2 apples, peeled, cored, and cubed
- 4 cups vegetable broth
- 1 teaspoon ground cinnamon
- 1/2 teaspoon ground nutmeg
- Salt and pepper to taste

Instructions:

1. Heat olive oil in a large pot over medium heat. Add diced onion and cook until softened, about 5 minutes.
2. Add minced garlic and cook for another minute.
3. Add cubed butternut squash, cubed apples, vegetable broth, ground

cinnamon, and ground nutmeg. Bring
to a boil.

4. Reduce heat to low and simmer for
   20-25 minutes, or until squash and
   apples are tender.

5. Use an immersion blender to blend
   the soup until smooth. Alternatively,
   transfer the soup to a blender and
   blend until smooth.

6. Season with salt and pepper to taste
   before serving.

Nutritional Information (per serving):

- Calories: 180
- Protein: 2g
- Carbohydrates: 30g
- Fat: 7g
- Fiber: 7g
- Sugar: 12g

1. Berry Blast Smoothie

Ingredients:

- 1 cup mixed berries (strawberries, blueberries, raspberries)
- 1 ripe banana
- 1/2 cup Greek yogurt
- 1/2 cup almond milk (or any milk of your choice)
- 1 tablespoon honey (optional)
- Ice cubes (optional)

Instructions:

1. Place all ingredients in a blender.
2. Blend until smooth.
3. If desired, add ice cubes and blend again until desired consistency is reached.

4. Pour into glasses and serve immediately.

Nutritional Information (per serving):

- Calories: 150
- Protein: 6g
- Carbohydrates: 30g
- Fat: 1g
- Fiber: 5g
- Sugar: 20g

2. Green Power Smoothie

Ingredients:

- 1 cup spinach
- 1/2 ripe avocado
- 1/2 cup pineapple chunks
- 1/2 banana
- 1/2 cup coconut water
- Juice of 1/2 lime
- Ice cubes (optional)

Instructions:

1. Place all ingredients in a blender.
2. Blend until smooth.
3. If desired, add ice cubes and blend again until desired consistency is reached.
4. Pour into glasses and serve immediately.

Nutritional Information (per serving):

- Calories: 180
- Protein: 3g
- Carbohydrates: 25g
- Fat: 9g
- Fiber: 7g
- Sugar: 15g

3. Tropical Paradise Smoothie

Ingredients:

- 1/2 cup frozen mango chunks
- 1/2 cup frozen pineapple chunks
- 1/2 ripe banana
- 1/2 cup coconut milk
- 1/4 cup Greek yogurt
- 1 tablespoon honey (optional)
- Ice cubes (optional)

Instructions:

1. Place all ingredients in a blender.
2. Blend until smooth.
3. If desired, add ice cubes and blend again until desired consistency is reached.
4. Pour into glasses and serve immediately.

Nutritional Information (per serving):

- Calories: 200
- Protein: 5g
- Carbohydrates: 35g

- Fat: 6g
- Fiber: 4g
- Sugar: 25g

4. Chocolate Peanut Butter Protein Shake

Ingredients:

- 1 cup almond milk (or any milk of your choice)
- 1 scoop chocolate protein powder
- 1 tablespoon cocoa powder
- 1 tablespoon peanut butter
- 1/2 ripe banana
- Ice cubes (optional)

Instructions:

1. Place all ingredients in a blender.
2. Blend until smooth.

3. If desired, add ice cubes and blend again until desired consistency is reached.
4. Pour into glasses and serve immediately.

Nutritional Information (per serving):

- Calories: 280
- Protein: 25g
- Carbohydrates: 25g
- Fat: 10g
- Fiber: 5g
- Sugar: 10g

5. Banana Oatmeal Breakfast Smoothie

Ingredients:

- 1 ripe banana
- 1/2 cup rolled oats

- 1/2 cup Greek yogurt
- 1/2 cup almond milk (or any milk of your choice)
- 1 tablespoon honey (optional)
- 1/2 teaspoon vanilla extract
- Pinch of cinnamon
- Ice cubes (optional)

Instructions:

1. Place all ingredients in a blender.
2. Blend until smooth.
3. If desired, add ice cubes and blend again until desired consistency is reached.
4. Pour into glasses and serve immediately.

Nutritional Information (per serving):

- Calories: 250
- Protein: 10g
- Carbohydrates: 45g

- Fat: 4g
- Fiber: 6g
- Sugar: 18g

1. Quinoa Stuffed Bell Peppers

Ingredients:

- 4 large bell peppers, halved and seeds removed
- 1 cup quinoa, cooked according to package instructions
- 1 can (15 oz) black beans, drained and rinsed
- 1 cup corn kernels
- 1 cup diced tomatoes
- 1/2 cup diced red onion
- 1/4 cup chopped fresh cilantro
- 1 teaspoon ground cumin
- 1 teaspoon chili powder
- Salt and pepper to taste

- Optional toppings: avocado slices, salsa, vegan sour cream

Instructions:

1. Preheat the oven to 375°F (190°C). Arrange bell pepper halves in a baking dish.
2. In a large bowl, combine cooked quinoa, black beans, corn, diced tomatoes, diced red onion, chopped cilantro, ground cumin, chili powder, salt, and pepper.
3. Spoon the quinoa mixture into each bell pepper half until they are filled.
4. Cover the baking dish with foil and bake for 25-30 minutes, or until the peppers are tender.
5. Remove from the oven and serve hot with optional toppings.

Nutritional Information (per serving, without toppings):

- Calories: 250
- Protein: 10g
- Carbohydrates: 45g
- Fat: 2g
- Fiber: 10g
- Sugar: 6g

2. Vegetable Stir-Fry with Tofu

Ingredients:

- 1 block (14 oz) extra firm tofu, pressed and cubed
- 2 tablespoons soy sauce
- 1 tablespoon sesame oil
- 1 tablespoon cornstarch
- 1 tablespoon vegetable oil
- 2 cloves garlic, minced
- 1 tablespoon grated ginger

- 2 cups mixed vegetables (bell peppers, broccoli, carrots, snap peas)
- Cooked brown rice or quinoa, for serving

Instructions:

1. In a bowl, toss cubed tofu with soy sauce, sesame oil, and cornstarch until evenly coated.
2. Heat vegetable oil in a large skillet over medium-high heat. Add minced garlic and grated ginger, and cook for 1 minute.
3. Add tofu cubes to the skillet and cook until golden brown on all sides, about 5-7 minutes. Remove from skillet and set aside.
4. In the same skillet, add mixed vegetables and stir-fry until tender-crisp, about 5 minutes.
5. Return tofu to the skillet and toss everything together until heated through.

6. Serve hot over cooked brown rice or quinoa.

Nutritional Information (per serving, tofu and vegetables only):

- Calories: 300
- Protein: 20g
- Carbohydrates: 25g
- Fat: 15g
- Fiber: 6g
- Sugar: 6g

3. Coconut Curry Lentil Soup

Ingredients:

- 1 tablespoon coconut oil
- 1 onion, diced
- 2 cloves garlic, minced
- 1 tablespoon grated ginger
- 2 carrots, diced
- 1 sweet potato, peeled and diced

- 1 cup red lentils, rinsed
- 4 cups vegetable broth
- 1 can (14 oz) coconut milk
- 2 tablespoons curry powder
- Salt and pepper to taste
- Fresh cilantro, for garnish

Instructions:

1. Heat coconut oil in a large pot over medium heat. Add diced onion, minced garlic, and grated ginger. Cook until softened, about 5 minutes.
2. Add diced carrots and sweet potato to the pot and cook for another 5 minutes.
3. Stir in red lentils, vegetable broth, coconut milk, and curry powder. Bring to a boil, then reduce heat to low and simmer for 20-25 minutes, or until lentils and vegetables are tender.
4. Season with salt and pepper to taste.
5. Serve hot, garnished with fresh cilantro.

Nutritional Information (per serving):

- Calories: 350
- Protein: 15g
- Carbohydrates: 45g
- Fat: 15g
- Fiber: 10g
- Sugar: 8g

4. Chickpea and Vegetable Curry

Ingredients:

- 1 tablespoon coconut oil
- 1 onion, diced
- 2 cloves garlic, minced
- 1 tablespoon grated ginger
- 2 cups cauliflower florets
- 1 can (15 oz) chickpeas, drained and rinsed
- 1 can (14 oz) diced tomatoes
- 1 can (14 oz) coconut milk
- 2 tablespoons curry powder
- Salt and pepper to taste

- Fresh cilantro, for garnish

Instructions:

1. Heat coconut oil in a large skillet over medium heat. Add diced onion, minced garlic, and grated ginger. Cook until softened, about 5 minutes.
2. Add cauliflower florets to the skillet and cook for another 5 minutes.
3. Stir in chickpeas, diced tomatoes, coconut milk, and curry powder. Bring to a simmer and cook for 15-20 minutes, or until cauliflower is tender.
4. Season with salt and pepper to taste.
5. Serve hot, garnished with fresh cilantro.

Nutritional Information (per serving):

- Calories: 300
- Protein: 10g
- Carbohydrates: 35g

- Fat: 15g
- Fiber: 10g
- Sugar: 8g

5. **Vegetable and Lentil Curry**

Ingredients:

- 1 tablespoon olive oil
- 1 onion, diced
- 2 cloves garlic, minced
- 1 tablespoon grated ginger
- 2 carrots, diced
- 2 celery stalks, diced
- 1 bell pepper, diced
- 1 cup dried green lentils, rinsed
- 1 can (14 oz) diced tomatoes
- 2 cups vegetable broth
- 2 tablespoons curry powder
- Salt and pepper to taste
- Fresh cilantro, for garnish

Instructions:

1. Heat olive oil in a large pot over medium heat. Add diced onion, minced garlic, and grated ginger. Cook until softened, about 5 minutes.
2. Add diced carrots, diced celery, and diced bell pepper to the pot and cook for another 5 minutes.
3. Stir in dried green lentils, diced tomatoes, vegetable broth, and curry powder. Bring to a boil, then reduce heat to low and simmer for 20-25 minutes, or until lentils are tender.
4. Season with salt and pepper to taste.
5. Serve hot, garnished with fresh cilantro.

Nutritional Information (per serving):

- Calories: 250
- Protein: 12g
- Carbohydrates: 40g
- Fat: 3g

- Fiber: 15g
- Sugar: 8g

BONUS

1. Grilled Lemon Herb Chicken with Asparagus

Ingredients:

- 4 boneless, skinless chicken breasts
- 1 bunch asparagus, trimmed
- 2 tablespoons olive oil
- 2 cloves garlic, minced
- Zest and juice of 1 lemon
- 1 tablespoon chopped fresh herbs (such as rosemary, thyme, or parsley)
- Salt and pepper to taste

Instructions:

1. Preheat grill to medium-high heat.

2. In a small bowl, whisk together olive oil, minced garlic, lemon zest, lemon juice, chopped herbs, salt, and pepper.
3. Place chicken breasts and asparagus on the grill. Brush with the lemon herb marinade.
4. Grill chicken for 6-8 minutes per side, or until cooked through. Grill asparagus for 4-5 minutes, or until tender-crisp.
5. Remove chicken and asparagus from the grill and serve hot.

Nutritional Information (per serving):

- Calories: 250
- Protein: 30g
- Carbohydrates: 5g
- Fat: 12g
- Fiber: 2g
- Sugar: 2g

2. Salmon and Quinoa Salad

Ingredients:

- 2 salmon fillets
- 1 cup cooked quinoa
- 2 cups mixed salad greens
- 1 cup cherry tomatoes, halved
- 1/2 cucumber, sliced
- 1/4 cup sliced red onion
- 2 tablespoons balsamic vinaigrette
- Salt and pepper to taste

Instructions:

1. Season salmon fillets with salt and pepper. Cook salmon in a skillet over medium-high heat for 3-4 minutes per side, or until cooked through.
2. In a large bowl, combine cooked quinoa, mixed salad greens, cherry tomatoes, sliced cucumber, and sliced red onion.
3. Drizzle with balsamic vinaigrette and toss to combine.

4. Divide the salad onto plates and top with cooked salmon fillets.
5. Serve immediately.

Nutritional Information (per serving):

- Calories: 350
- Protein: 30g
- Carbohydrates: 25g
- Fat: 15g
- Fiber: 5g
- Sugar: 5g

3. Turkey and Vegetable Lettuce Wraps

Ingredients:

- 1 lb ground turkey
- 1 tablespoon olive oil
- 1 onion, diced
- 2 cloves garlic, minced

- 1 bell pepper, diced
- 1 zucchini, diced
- 1 carrot, grated
- 1 teaspoon ground cumin
- 1 teaspoon chili powder
- Salt and pepper to taste
- Iceberg or butter lettuce leaves, for wrapping

Instructions:

1. Heat olive oil in a skillet over medium heat. Add diced onion and minced garlic, and cook until softened.
2. Add ground turkey to the skillet and cook until browned.
3. Add diced bell pepper, diced zucchini, grated carrot, ground cumin, chili powder, salt, and pepper. Cook until vegetables are tender.
4. Spoon the turkey and vegetable mixture onto lettuce leaves.
5. Roll up the lettuce leaves and secure with toothpicks, if needed.

6. Serve immediately.

Nutritional Information (per serving):

- Calories: 200
- Protein: 20g
- Carbohydrates: 10g
- Fat: 8g
- Fiber: 3g
- Sugar: 5g

4. Vegetable and Tofu Stir-Fry

Ingredients:

- 1 tablespoon sesame oil
- 1 block (14 oz) extra firm tofu, pressed and cubed
- 2 cups mixed vegetables (broccoli, bell peppers, snap peas, carrots)
- 2 cloves garlic, minced
- 2 tablespoons soy sauce
- 1 tablespoon hoisin sauce

- 1 teaspoon cornstarch
- Cooked brown rice, for serving

Instructions:

1. Heat sesame oil in a large skillet over medium-high heat. Add cubed tofu and cook until golden brown on all sides.
2. Add mixed vegetables and minced garlic to the skillet. Stir-fry until vegetables are tender-crisp.
3. In a small bowl, whisk together soy sauce, hoisin sauce, and cornstarch. Pour the sauce over the tofu and vegetables.
4. Cook for another 2-3 minutes, until the sauce has thickened.
5. Serve hot over cooked brown rice.

Nutritional Information (per serving):

- Calories: 300

- Protein: 20g
- Carbohydrates: 30g
- Fat: 12g
- Fiber: 6g
- Sugar: 5g

5. Mediterranean Chickpea Salad

Ingredients:

- 2 cups cooked chickpeas (or 1 can, drained and rinsed)
- 1 cucumber, diced
- 1 bell pepper, diced
- 1/2 red onion, thinly sliced
- 1/4 cup Kalamata olives, sliced
- 1/4 cup crumbled feta cheese (optional)
- 2 tablespoons chopped fresh parsley
- Juice of 1 lemon
- 2 tablespoons olive oil
- Salt and pepper to taste

Instructions:

1. In a large bowl, combine cooked chickpeas, diced cucumber, diced bell pepper, sliced red onion, sliced Kalamata olives, crumbled feta cheese (if using), and chopped fresh parsley.
2. Drizzle with lemon juice and olive oil. Season with salt and pepper to taste.
3. Toss to combine all ingredients.
4. Serve chilled or at room temperature.

Nutritional Information (per serving, without feta cheese):

- Calories: 250
- Protein: 10g
- Carbohydrates: 30g
- Fat: 10g
- Fiber: 8g
- Sugar: 5g

BONUS

1. **Green Detox Juice**

Ingredients:

- 1 cucumber
- 2 celery stalks
- 1 green apple
- 1 cup spinach
- 1 lemon (peeled)
- 1-inch piece of ginger
- 1 cup water

Instructions:

1. Wash all the ingredients thoroughly.
2. Cut the cucumber, celery, apple, and lemon into chunks.
3. Add all ingredients to a blender along with the water.
4. Blend until smooth.

5. Strain the juice through a fine mesh sieve or cheesecloth to remove the pulp, if desired.
6. Serve immediately.

Nutritional Information (per serving):

- Calories: 80
- Protein: 1g
- Carbohydrates: 19g
- Fat: 0.5g
- Fiber: 4g
- Sugar: 10g

2. Berry Smoothie

Ingredients:

- 1 cup mixed berries (strawberries, blueberries, raspberries)
- 1/2 cup unsweetened almond milk
- 1/2 cup Greek yogurt
- 1 tablespoon chia seeds

- 1 teaspoon honey (optional)
- Ice cubes (optional)

Instructions:

1. Add all ingredients to a blender.
2. Blend until smooth.
3. Add ice cubes if desired and blend again until desired consistency is reached.
4. Serve immediately.

Nutritional Information (per serving):

- Calories: 140
- Protein: 8g
- Carbohydrates: 20g
- Fat: 4g
- Fiber: 6g
- Sugar: 12g

3. Turmeric Golden Milk

Ingredients:

- 1 cup unsweetened almond milk
- 1 teaspoon ground turmeric
- 1/4 teaspoon ground ginger
- 1/4 teaspoon ground cinnamon
- 1 teaspoon maple syrup or honey (optional)
- Pinch of black pepper

Instructions:

1. Heat the almond milk in a small saucepan over medium heat.
2. Add the turmeric, ginger, cinnamon, and black pepper. Whisk to combine.
3. Simmer for 5 minutes, stirring occasionally.
4. If using, stir in maple syrup or honey.
5. Pour into a mug and serve warm.

Nutritional Information (per serving):

- Calories: 60

- Protein: 1g
- Carbohydrates: 8g
- Fat: 3g
- Fiber: 1g
- Sugar: 5g

4. Matcha Latte

Ingredients:

- 1 teaspoon matcha green tea powder
- 1/4 cup hot water (not boiling)
- 3/4 cup unsweetened almond milk
- 1 teaspoon honey or maple syrup (optional)

Instructions:

1. Sift the matcha powder into a mug to remove any clumps.
2. Add the hot water and whisk vigorously until the matcha is fully dissolved and frothy.

3. Heat the almond milk in a small saucepan or microwave until warm.
4. Froth the almond milk using a milk frother or whisk.
5. Pour the frothed almond milk into the matcha mixture.
6. Stir in honey or maple syrup if desired.
7. Serve immediately.

Nutritional Information (per serving):

- Calories: 50
- Protein: 1g
- Carbohydrates: 7g
- Fat: 2g
- Fiber: 1g
- Sugar: 5g

5. Cucumber Mint Water

Ingredients:

- 1 cucumber, thinly sliced
- 1 lemon, thinly sliced
- 10 fresh mint leaves
- 8 cups water
- Ice cubes (optional)

Instructions:

1. In a large pitcher, combine cucumber slices, lemon slices, and mint leaves.
2. Add the water and stir to combine.
3. Refrigerate for at least 2 hours to allow flavors to infuse.
4. Serve chilled, with ice cubes if desired.

Nutritional Information (per serving):

- Calories: 5
- Protein: 0g
- Carbohydrates: 1g
- Fat: 0g
- Fiber: 0g
- Sugar: 0g

Day 1

Breakfast: Berry Blast Smoothie

- Ingredients: 1 cup mixed berries, 1 banana, 1/2 cup Greek yogurt, 1/2 cup almond milk, 1 tbsp honey (optional)
- Instructions: Blend all ingredients until smooth. Serve immediately.
- Nutritional Information: 150 calories, 6g protein, 30g carbs, 1g fat, 5g fiber, 20g sugar

Lunch: Quinoa Stuffed Bell Peppers

- Ingredients: 4 bell peppers, 1 cup quinoa, 1 can black beans, 1 cup corn, 1 cup diced tomatoes, 1/2 cup red

onion, 1/4 cup cilantro, 1 tsp cumin, 1 tsp chili powder, salt, pepper
- Instructions: Cook quinoa. Mix with beans, corn, tomatoes, onion, cilantro, spices. Stuff peppers and bake at 375°F for 25-30 minutes.
- Nutritional Information: 250 calories, 10g protein, 45g carbs, 2g fat, 10g fiber, 6g sugar

Dinner: Grilled Lemon Herb Chicken with Asparagus

- Ingredients: 4 chicken breasts, 1 bunch asparagus, 2 tbsp olive oil, 2 garlic cloves, zest/juice of 1 lemon, 1 tbsp herbs, salt, pepper
- Instructions: Marinate chicken and asparagus with oil, garlic, lemon, herbs. Grill chicken 6-8 min per side, asparagus 4-5 min.

- Nutritional Information: 250 calories, 30g protein, 5g carbs, 12g fat, 2g fiber, 2g sugar

Snack: Apple Slices with Almond Butter

- Ingredients: 1 apple, 2 tbsp almond butter
- Nutritional Information: 190 calories, 4g protein, 26g carbs, 9g fat, 5g fiber, 19g sugar

Day 2

Breakfast: Green Power Smoothie

- Ingredients: 1 cup spinach, 1/2 avocado, 1/2 cup pineapple, 1/2 banana, 1/2 cup coconut water, juice of 1/2 lime
- Instructions: Blend all ingredients until smooth. Serve immediately.

- Nutritional Information: 180 calories, 3g protein, 25g carbs, 9g fat, 7g fiber, 15g sugar

Lunch: Salmon and Quinoa Salad

- Ingredients: 2 salmon fillets, 1 cup quinoa, 2 cups greens, 1 cup cherry tomatoes, 1/2 cucumber, 1/4 cup red onion, 2 tbsp balsamic vinaigrette
- Instructions: Cook salmon and quinoa. Mix quinoa, greens, tomatoes, cucumber, onion, vinaigrette. Top with salmon.
- Nutritional Information: 350 calories, 30g protein, 25g carbs, 15g fat, 5g fiber, 5g sugar

Dinner: Vegetable and Lentil Curry

- Ingredients: 1 tbsp olive oil, 1 onion, 2 garlic cloves, 1 tbsp ginger, 2 carrots, 2 celery stalks, 1 bell pepper, 1 cup lentils, 1 can tomatoes, 2 cups broth, 2 tbsp curry powder

- Instructions: Sauté onion, garlic, ginger. Add vegetables, lentils, tomatoes, broth, curry. Simmer 20-25 minutes.
- Nutritional Information: 250 calories, 12g protein, 40g carbs, 3g fat, 15g fiber, 8g sugar

Snack: Carrot Sticks with Hummus

- Ingredients: 1 cup carrot sticks, 1/4 cup hummus
- Nutritional Information: 150 calories, 4g protein, 16g carbs, 8g fat, 5g fiber, 5g sugar

Day 3

Breakfast: Banana Oatmeal Breakfast Smoothie

- Ingredients: 1 banana, 1/2 cup oats, 1/2 cup Greek yogurt, 1/2 cup almond milk, 1 tbsp honey, 1/2 tsp vanilla, pinch of cinnamon
- Instructions: Blend all ingredients until smooth. Serve immediately.
- Nutritional Information: 250 calories, 10g protein, 45g carbs, 4g fat, 6g fiber, 18g sugar

Lunch: Chickpea and Vegetable Curry

- Ingredients: 1 tbsp coconut oil, 1 onion, 2 garlic cloves, 1 tbsp ginger, 2 cups cauliflower, 1 can chickpeas, 1 can tomatoes, 1 can coconut milk, 2 tbsp curry powder
- Instructions: Sauté onion, garlic, ginger. Add cauliflower, chickpeas, tomatoes, coconut milk, curry. Simmer 15-20 minutes.
- Nutritional Information: 300 calories, 10g protein, 35g carbs, 15g fat, 10g fiber, 8g sugar

Dinner: Turkey and Vegetable Lettuce Wraps

- Ingredients: 1 lb ground turkey, 1 tbsp olive oil, 1 onion, 2 garlic cloves, 1 bell pepper, 1 zucchini, 1 carrot, 1 tsp cumin, 1 tsp chili powder, salt, pepper, lettuce leaves
- Instructions: Sauté onion, garlic, turkey. Add vegetables, spices. Cook until tender. Serve in lettuce leaves.
- Nutritional Information: 200 calories, 20g protein, 10g carbs, 8g fat, 3g fiber, 5g sugar

Snack: Mixed Nuts

- Ingredients: 1/4 cup mixed nuts
- Nutritional Information: 200 calories, 6g protein, 7g carbs, 18g fat, 3g fiber, 2g sugar

Day 4

Breakfast: Tropical Paradise Smoothie

- Ingredients: 1/2 cup mango, 1/2 cup pineapple, 1/2 banana, 1/2 cup coconut milk, 1/4 cup Greek yogurt, 1 tbsp honey
- Instructions: Blend all ingredients until smooth. Serve immediately.
- Nutritional Information: 200 calories, 5g protein, 35g carbs, 6g fat, 4g fiber, 25g sugar

Lunch: Mediterranean Chickpea Salad

- Ingredients: 2 cups chickpeas, 1 cucumber, 1 bell pepper, 1/2 red onion, 1/4 cup olives, 1/4 cup feta, 2 tbsp parsley, juice of 1 lemon, 2 tbsp olive oil, salt, pepper
- Instructions: Mix all ingredients. Serve chilled or at room temperature.
- Nutritional Information: 250 calories, 10g protein, 30g carbs, 10g fat, 8g fiber, 5g sugar

Dinner: Vegetable and Tofu Stir-Fry

- Ingredients: 1 tbsp sesame oil, 1 block tofu, 2 cups mixed vegetables, 2 garlic cloves, 2 tbsp soy sauce, 1 tbsp hoisin sauce, 1 tsp cornstarch, brown rice
- Instructions: Sauté tofu in sesame oil until golden. Add vegetables, garlic. Mix soy sauce, hoisin, cornstarch. Add to pan, cook until thickened. Serve over rice.
- Nutritional Information: 300 calories, 20g protein, 30g carbs, 12g fat, 6g fiber, 5g sugar

Snack: Fresh Fruit Salad

- Ingredients: 1 cup mixed fresh fruits (berries, melons, citrus)
- Nutritional Information: 100 calories, 1g protein, 25g carbs, 0g fat, 5g fiber, 20g sugar

Day 5

Breakfast: Matcha Latte

- Ingredients: 1 tsp matcha, 1/4 cup hot water, 3/4 cup almond milk, 1 tsp honey
- Instructions: Dissolve matcha in hot water. Froth almond milk. Mix and serve warm.
- Nutritional Information: 50 calories, 1g protein, 7g carbs, 2g fat, 1g fiber, 5g sugar

Lunch: Lentil and Vegetable Soup

- Ingredients: 1 tbsp olive oil, 1 onion, 2 garlic cloves, 1 carrot, 2 celery stalks, 1 bell pepper, 1 cup lentils, 1 can tomatoes, 4 cups broth, 1 tsp thyme
- Instructions: Sauté onion, garlic. Add vegetables, lentils, tomatoes, broth, thyme. Simmer 20-25 minutes.

- Nutritional Information: 250 calories, 12g protein, 40g carbs, 3g fat, 15g fiber, 8g sugar

Dinner: Baked Cod with Sweet Potato Fries

- Ingredients: 4 cod fillets, 2 sweet potatoes, 2 tbsp olive oil, 1 tsp paprika, 1 tsp garlic powder, salt, pepper, lemon wedges
- Instructions: Preheat oven to 400°F. Slice sweet potatoes into fries, toss with 1 tbsp olive oil, paprika, garlic powder, salt, and pepper. Bake for 25-30 minutes. Season cod fillets with salt, pepper, and remaining olive oil. Bake for 15-20 minutes. Serve with lemon wedges.
- Nutritional Information: 350 calories, 25g protein, 30g carbs, 12g fat, 5g fiber, 5g sugar

Snack: Greek Yogurt with Berries

- Ingredients: 1/2 cup Greek yogurt, 1/2 cup mixed berries, 1 tsp honey
- Nutritional Information: 100 calories, 10g protein, 15g carbs, 0g fat, 2g fiber, 12g sugar

Day 6

Breakfast: Chia Seed Pudding

- Ingredients: 1/4 cup chia seeds, 1 cup almond milk, 1 tbsp honey, 1/2 tsp vanilla extract, 1/4 cup fresh berries
- Instructions: Mix chia seeds, almond milk, honey, and vanilla in a bowl. Refrigerate overnight. Top with berries before serving.
- Nutritional Information: 200 calories, 5g protein, 25g carbs, 10g fat, 10g fiber, 12g sugar

Lunch: Spinach and Quinoa Salad

- Ingredients: 1 cup cooked quinoa, 2 cups spinach, 1/2 cup cherry tomatoes, 1/2 cucumber, 1/4 cup feta cheese, 2 tbsp balsamic vinaigrette
- Instructions: Mix all ingredients in a large bowl. Serve immediately.
- Nutritional Information: 250 calories, 10g protein, 30g carbs, 10g fat, 6g fiber, 5g sugar

Dinner: Shrimp Stir-Fry

- Ingredients: 1 lb shrimp, 2 cups mixed vegetables, 2 tbsp soy sauce, 1 tbsp hoisin sauce, 1 tbsp sesame oil, 2 cloves garlic, 1 tsp ginger
- Instructions: Sauté garlic and ginger in sesame oil. Add shrimp and cook until pink. Add vegetables and sauces. Cook until vegetables are tender.

- Nutritional Information: 300 calories, 25g protein, 20g carbs, 10g fat, 5g fiber, 6g sugar

Snack: Celery Sticks with Peanut Butter

- Ingredients: 1 cup celery sticks, 2 tbsp peanut butter
- Nutritional Information: 150 calories, 5g protein, 12g carbs, 10g fat, 3g fiber, 5g sugar

Day 7

Breakfast: Oatmeal with Banana and Almonds

- Ingredients: 1/2 cup oats, 1 cup almond milk, 1 banana, 1 tbsp sliced almonds, 1 tsp honey
- Instructions: Cook oats in almond milk. Top with sliced banana, almonds, and honey. Serve warm.

- Nutritional Information: 250 calories, 6g protein, 45g carbs, 8g fat, 6g fiber, 15g sugar

Lunch: Turkey and Avocado Wrap

- Ingredients: 1 whole wheat wrap, 4 oz turkey breast, 1/2 avocado, 1/4 cup lettuce, 1/4 cup tomatoes, 1 tbsp mustard
- Instructions: Spread mustard on the wrap. Add turkey, avocado, lettuce, and tomatoes. Roll up and serve.
- Nutritional Information: 300 calories, 20g protein, 30g carbs, 12g fat, 6g fiber, 4g sugar

Dinner: Grilled Chicken with Mixed Veggies

- Ingredients: 4 chicken breasts, 2 cups broccoli, 1 cup bell peppers, 1 cup zucchini, 2 tbsp olive oil, 1 tbsp Italian seasoning, salt, pepper

- Instructions: Marinate chicken in olive oil, Italian seasoning, salt, and pepper. Grill chicken until cooked through. Sauté vegetables in olive oil until tender. Serve together.
- Nutritional Information: 350 calories, 35g protein, 15g carbs, 15g fat, 6g fiber, 7g sugar

Snack: Cottage Cheese with Pineapple

- Ingredients: 1/2 cup cottage cheese, 1/2 cup pineapple chunks
- Nutritional Information: 100 calories, 10g protein, 15g carbs, 2g fat, 2g fiber, 12g sugar

Day 8

Breakfast: Avocado Toast with Poached Egg

Ingredients: 1 slice whole grain bread, 1/2 avocado, 1 poached egg, salt, pepper, red pepper flakes

Instructions: Toast the bread. Mash the avocado and spread on toast. Top with poached egg, salt, pepper, and red pepper flakes.

Nutritional Information: 250 calories, 10g protein, 20g carbs, 15g fat, 7g fiber, 2g sugar

Lunch: Chicken Caesar Salad

Ingredients: 4 cups romaine lettuce, 1 chicken breast (grilled), 1/4 cup parmesan cheese, 1/2 cup croutons, 2 tbsp Caesar dressing

Instructions: Slice the chicken breast. Toss lettuce, chicken, parmesan, and croutons with Caesar dressing.

Nutritional Information: 350 calories, 30g protein, 20g carbs, 18g fat, 5g fiber, 4g sugar

Dinner: Beef and Broccoli Stir-Fry

Ingredients: 1 lb beef strips, 2 cups broccoli florets, 1 bell pepper, 2 tbsp soy sauce, 1 tbsp hoisin sauce, 1 tbsp olive oil, 1 garlic clove, 1 tsp ginger

Instructions: Sauté garlic and ginger in olive oil. Add beef and cook until browned. Add broccoli, bell pepper, soy sauce, and hoisin sauce. Cook until vegetables are tender.

Nutritional Information: 400 calories, 30g protein, 20g carbs, 20g fat, 6g fiber, 7g sugar

Snack: Apple with Peanut Butter
Ingredients: 1 apple, 2 tbsp peanut butter
Nutritional Information: 200 calories, 4g protein, 30g carbs, 9g fat, 5g fiber, 19g sugar

Day 9

Breakfast: Greek Yogurt Parfait

Ingredients: 1 cup Greek yogurt, 1/2 cup granola, 1/2 cup mixed berries, 1 tbsp honey

Instructions: Layer yogurt, granola, and berries in a bowl or jar. Drizzle with honey.

Nutritional Information: 300 calories, 15g protein, 45g carbs, 8g fat, 6g fiber, 22g sugar

Lunch: Tuna Salad Wrap

Ingredients: 1 can tuna, 2 tbsp Greek yogurt, 1 tbsp mayonnaise, 1 celery stalk, 1/4 red onion, 1 tsp Dijon mustard, 1 whole wheat wrap, lettuce leaves

Instructions: Mix tuna, yogurt, mayonnaise, diced celery, onion, and mustard. Spread on wrap, top with lettuce, and roll up.

Nutritional Information: 250 calories, 20g protein, 30g carbs, 8g fat, 5g fiber, 4g sugar

Dinner: Spaghetti Squash with Marinara Sauce

Ingredients: 1 spaghetti squash, 2 cups marinara sauce, 1/4 cup parmesan cheese, 1 tbsp olive oil, 1 garlic clove, salt, pepper

Instructions: Cut spaghetti squash in half, remove seeds, and bake at 400°F for 40 minutes. Scrape out strands. Sauté garlic in olive oil, add marinara sauce, and heat. Serve sauce over squash, topped with parmesan.

Nutritional Information: 300 calories, 10g protein, 35g carbs, 12g fat, 6g fiber, 12g sugar
Snack: Mixed Berries

Ingredients: 1 cup mixed berries (strawberries, blueberries, raspberries)
Nutritional Information: 70 calories, 1g protein, 18g carbs, 0g fat, 6g fiber, 12g sugar

Day 10

Breakfast: Peanut Butter Banana Smoothie

Ingredients: 1 banana, 1 tbsp peanut butter, 1/2 cup Greek yogurt, 1/2 cup almond milk, 1 tbsp honey

Instructions: Blend all ingredients until smooth. Serve immediately.

Nutritional Information: 250 calories, 10g protein, 40g carbs, 8g fat, 4g fiber, 22g sugar

Lunch: Quinoa and Black Bean Salad

Ingredients: 1 cup cooked quinoa, 1 can black beans, 1 cup corn, 1 red bell pepper,

1/4 cup red onion, 1/4 cup cilantro, juice of 1 lime, 2 tbsp olive oil, salt, pepper

Instructions: Mix all ingredients in a large bowl. Serve chilled or at room temperature.

Nutritional Information: 300 calories, 10g protein, 45g carbs, 8g fat, 10g fiber, 6g sugar

Dinner: Baked Salmon with Asparagus

Ingredients: 4 salmon fillets, 1 bunch asparagus, 2 tbsp olive oil, 2 garlic cloves, zest/juice of 1 lemon, salt, pepper

Instructions: Preheat oven to 400°F. Place salmon and asparagus on a baking sheet. Drizzle with olive oil, lemon juice, and season with salt and pepper. Bake for 15-20 minutes.

Nutritional Information: 350 calories, 30g protein, 10g carbs, 20g fat, 5g fiber, 4g sugar

Snack: Cottage Cheese with Pineapple

Ingredients: 1/2 cup cottage cheese, 1/2 cup pineapple chunks
Nutritional Information: 100 calories, 10g protein, 15g carbs, 2g fat, 2g fiber, 12g sugar

Day 11

Breakfast: Overnight Oats

Ingredients: 1/2 cup oats, 1/2 cup almond milk, 1/4 cup Greek yogurt, 1 tbsp chia seeds, 1 tbsp honey, 1/2 cup blueberries

Instructions: Mix oats, almond milk, yogurt, chia seeds, and honey in a jar. Refrigerate overnight. Top with blueberries before serving.

Nutritional Information: 300 calories, 10g protein, 50g carbs, 8g fat, 10g fiber, 20g sugar

Lunch: Hummus and Veggie Wrap

Ingredients: 1 whole wheat wrap, 1/2 cup hummus, 1/2 cucumber, 1/2 bell pepper, 1/4 cup shredded carrots, 1/4 cup spinach

Instructions: Spread hummus on the wrap. Add sliced vegetables and spinach. Roll up and serve.

Nutritional Information: 250 calories, 7g protein, 35g carbs, 10g fat, 8g fiber, 5g sugar

Dinner: Chicken and Vegetable Skewers

Ingredients: 1 lb chicken breast, 1 bell pepper, 1 zucchini, 1 red onion, 1/4 cup olive oil, 2 tbsp soy sauce, 1 tbsp lemon juice, 1 tsp garlic powder, 1 tsp paprika

Instructions: Cut chicken and vegetables into chunks. Marinate in olive oil, soy sauce, lemon juice, garlic powder, and paprika.

Thread onto skewers and grill until cooked through.

Nutritional Information: 300 calories, 30g protein, 12g carbs, 15g fat, 4g fiber, 6g sugar

Snack: Carrot Sticks with Hummus
Ingredients: 1 cup carrot sticks, 1/4 cup hummus

Nutritional Information: 150 calories, 4g protein, 16g carbs, 8g fat, 5g fiber, 5g sugar

Day 12

Breakfast: Spinach and Mushroom Omelette

Ingredients: 3 eggs, 1/2 cup spinach, 1/4 cup mushrooms, 1 tbsp olive oil, salt, pepper

Instructions: Sauté spinach and mushrooms in olive oil. Beat eggs and pour into the pan. Cook until set. Season with salt and pepper.

Nutritional Information: 250 calories, 18g protein, 5g carbs, 18g fat, 2g fiber, 2g sugar

Lunch: Lentil Soup

Ingredients: 1 tbsp olive oil, 1 onion, 2 garlic cloves, 1 carrot, 2 celery stalks, 1 cup lentils, 1 can tomatoes, 4 cups broth, 1 tsp thyme, salt, pepper

Instructions: Sauté onion, garlic, carrot, and celery in olive oil. Add lentils, tomatoes, broth, thyme, salt, and pepper. Simmer for 25-30 minutes.

Nutritional Information: 250 calories, 12g protein, 40g carbs,

Lunch: Lentil Soup (Continued)

Nutritional Information: 250 calories, 12g protein, 40g carbs, 5g fat, 15g fiber, 8g sugar

Dinner: Stuffed Bell Peppers

Ingredients: 4 bell peppers, 1 lb ground turkey, 1 cup quinoa (cooked), 1 can diced tomatoes, 1/2 onion, 1 tbsp olive oil, 1 tsp cumin, 1 tsp paprika, salt, pepper

Instructions: Preheat oven to 375°F. Sauté onion in olive oil, add ground turkey and cook until browned. Add cooked quinoa, diced tomatoes, cumin, paprika, salt, and pepper. Cut tops off bell peppers and remove seeds. Stuff peppers with mixture and place in a baking dish. Bake for 30 minutes.

Nutritional Information: 300 calories, 25g protein, 30g carbs, 10g fat, 6g fiber, 8g sugar

Snack: Almonds

Ingredients: 1/4 cup raw almonds

Nutritional Information: 200 calories, 6g protein, 7g carbs, 18g fat, 4g fiber, 2g sugar

Day 13

Breakfast: Berry Smoothie Bowl

Ingredients: 1 cup mixed berries, 1 banana, 1/2 cup Greek yogurt, 1/2 cup almond milk, 1 tbsp chia seeds, 1 tbsp honey

Instructions: Blend berries, banana, yogurt, almond milk, and honey until smooth. Pour into a bowl and top with chia seeds.

Nutritional Information: 300 calories, 10g protein, 60g carbs, 6g fat, 10g fiber, 35g sugar

Lunch: Chickpea Salad

Ingredients: 1 can chickpeas (drained and rinsed), 1 cucumber, 1 cup cherry tomatoes,

1/4 red onion, 1/4 cup feta cheese, 2 tbsp olive oil, 1 tbsp lemon juice, salt, pepper

Instructions: Mix chickpeas, diced cucumber, halved cherry tomatoes, diced red onion, and crumbled feta. Dress with olive oil, lemon juice, salt, and pepper.

Nutritional Information: 300 calories, 10g protein, 30g carbs, 15g fat, 8g fiber, 5g sugar

Dinner: Zucchini Noodles with Pesto

Ingredients: 4 zucchinis (spiralized), 1/4 cup pesto, 1 tbsp olive oil, 1/4 cup cherry tomatoes, 1/4 cup parmesan cheese, salt, pepper

Instructions: Heat olive oil in a pan and sauté zucchini noodles for 2-3 minutes. Add pesto and cherry tomatoes, cook for another 2 minutes. Top with parmesan, salt, and pepper.

Nutritional Information: 250 calories, 10g protein, 12g carbs, 18g fat, 4g fiber, 6g sugar
Snack: Rice Cakes with Hummus

Ingredients: 2 rice cakes, 1/4 cup hummus
Nutritional Information: 150 calories, 4g protein, 20g carbs, 7g fat, 3g fiber, 2g sugar

Day 14

Breakfast: Fruit and Nut Oatmeal

Ingredients: 1/2 cup oats, 1 cup almond milk, 1/4 cup mixed nuts, 1/2 cup mixed fruit (such as berries or chopped apple), 1 tbsp honey

Instructions: Cook oats in almond milk. Top with mixed nuts, fruit, and honey. Serve warm.

Nutritional Information: 300 calories, 8g protein, 45g carbs, 12g fat, 6g fiber, 20g sugar

Lunch: Turkey and Avocado Salad

Ingredients: 4 cups mixed greens, 4 oz sliced turkey breast, 1/2 avocado, 1/4 cup cherry tomatoes, 1/4 cucumber, 2 tbsp olive oil, 1 tbsp balsamic vinegar, salt, pepper

Instructions: Mix greens, turkey, sliced avocado, halved cherry tomatoes, and sliced cucumber. Dress with olive oil, balsamic vinegar, salt, and pepper.

Nutritional Information: 300 calories, 20g protein, 15g carbs, 18g fat, 8g fiber, 4g sugar
Dinner: Vegetable Stir-Fry with Tofu

Ingredients: 1 block firm tofu, 2 cups broccoli, 1 red bell pepper, 1 cup snap peas, 1 carrot, 2 tbsp soy sauce, 1 tbsp sesame oil, 1 tbsp olive oil, 1 garlic clove, 1 tsp ginger

Instructions: Press tofu to remove excess water, then cut into cubes. Sauté garlic and ginger in olive oil. Add tofu and cook until browned. Add vegetables, soy sauce, and sesame oil. Cook until vegetables are tender.

Nutritional Information: 350 calories, 15g protein, 20g carbs, 22g fat, 6g fiber, 6g sugar

Snack: Sliced Bell Peppers with Guacamole
Ingredients: 1 bell pepper, 1/4 cup guacamole

Nutritional Information: 150 calories, 2g protein, 15g carbs, 10g fat, 6g fiber, 5g sugar

CONCLUSION

As you've learned throughout this book, the somatic diet is a powerful tool for regulating your nervous system and promoting overall well-being. By nourishing your body with whole, nutrient-dense foods and avoiding inflammatory triggers, you've taken a significant step towards calming dysregulation and restoring balance.

But the somatic diet is more than just a dietary approach – it's a lifestyle that embraces the interconnectedness of mind, body, and spirit. By tuning into your body's innate wisdom and honoring its needs, you've cultivated a deeper sense of self-awareness and self-compassion.

Through the practices of mindful eating, gentle movement, and stress management techniques, you've learned to navigate life's challenges with greater resilience and equanimity. The somatic diet has empowered you to become an active participant in your own healing journey, rather than a passive recipient of external remedies.

As you continue on this path, remember that the journey towards optimal nervous system regulation is not a linear one. There may be moments of setbacks and struggles, but with the tools and knowledge you've gained, you are better equipped to navigate these challenges with grace and patience.

Embrace the somatic diet as a way of life, a constant exploration of what nourishes your mind, body, and spirit. Celebrate the small victories and the moments of calm amidst the chaos. And above all, trust in the innate wisdom of your body, for it holds the key to unlocking a state of balanced nervous system regulation.

May this book serve as a constant reminder of the transformative power of the somatic diet, and may it inspire you to continue nurturing your body, mind, and spirit with intention and compassion. Your nervous system, and indeed your whole being, will thank you for this invaluable gift of self-care.

THE END